YOUR KNOWLEDGE HAS VALUE

- We will publish your bachelor's and
  master's thesis, essays and papers

- Your own eBook and book -
  sold worldwide in all relevant shops

- Earn money with each sale

Upload your text at www.GRIN.com
and publish for free

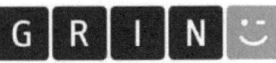

Bibliographic information published by the German National Library:

The German National Library lists this publication in the National Bibliography; detailed bibliographic data are available on the Internet at http://dnb.dnb.de .

Imprint:

Copyright © 2017 GRIN Verlag
Print and binding: Books on Demand GmbH, Norderstedt Germany
ISBN: 9783668740310

This book at GRIN:

https://www.grin.com/document/423939

Leon Kandoko

Ergonomic hazards on brick making industry. Case study of a brick company in Zimbabwe

GRIN Verlag

BINDURA UNIVERSITY OF SCIENCE EDUCATION

DEPARTMENT OF ENVIROMENTAL SCIENCE

AN ASSESSMENT OF ERGONOMIC HAZARDS IN BRICK MAKING INDUSTRY: CASE STUDY OF XY BRICKS ZIMBABWE.

KANDOKO LEON

A DISSERTATION SUBMITTED IN PARTIAL FULFILLMENT OF THE REQUIREMENTS OF THE BACHELOR OF ENVIRONMENTAL SCIENCE HONOURS DEGREE IN SAFETY HEALTH AND ENVIRONMRENTAL MANAGEMENT (BES-SHEM)

2017

DEDICATION

To my loving mother; Mrs. G Kandoko, the late Mr. C Kandoko, my best mentor; my father, my aunt; Mrs. S Moyo, my research supervisor, my young brother, friends and fellow students, this is for you.

ACKNOWLEDGEMENTS

I would like to first thank God for giving me strength, hope and endurance to be able to complete this study.

All gratitude is extended to University associates and accomplices who facilitated for the carrying out and completion of this study. Mrs L Mabhungu, my supervisor must be applauded for giving me guidance and assistance during the entire study. I would like to express my appreciation to XY Bricks[1] Zimbabwe that provided with the platform to conduct the research. Special thanks to my industrial attachment mentors Mrs K N. and Mr B C. and Ms N M. for their facility, technical guidance and support.

I would like to thank mother Mrs G Kandoko, my brother Mr I Kandoko and my friend Tinashe Malukula who supported me financially and emotionally during the whole course of this study. Thank you for encouraging me to be a hard worker and a center of excellence, l appreciate and love you most sincerely.

---

[1] Due to data protection reasons names have been changed by the editors.

ABSTRACT

The basic understanding of ergonomic hazards at work places is vital for the prevention of work related musculoskeletal related injuries. The study assessed the ergonomic hazards at XY Bricks. A cross sectional design was used to collect information on the hazards. The sample was drawn from five work sections covering from brick molding up to brick dispatch and these were; brick extruding, brick cutting, brick setting, brick packing and brick dispatching. The research was based on questionnaires and National Institute for Occupational Safety and Health (NOISH) inspection checklist for ergonomic factors as methods of gathering the required data. Total of 38 questionnaires were used to assess employees on common ergonomic hazards and ergonomic hazard awareness. The questionnaires were used to establish worker perceptions with regards to ergonomics. A total of 40 inspections were conducted using the National Institute for Occupational Safety and Health (NOISH) ergonomic checklist to identify the ergonomic hazards. Descriptive analysis was done using SPSS version 16.0 of 2007 to get frequency and percentiles. The results showed that the common ergonomic hazards were repetition, awkward postures, forceful motion, stationary work positions and vibration. The study found that employees are exposed to ergonomic hazards which include repetition, awkward postures, forceful motions, stationary working positions, vibration, work stress. From the results of the study it is evidenced that XY Bricks is not an ergonomically safe workplace. Therefore it will be important to implement ergonomics intervention at this brick manufacturing organization.

LIST OF FIGURES

LIST OF TABLES

---

[2] Due to data protection reasons this map has been deleted by the editors.

LIST OF ACRONYMS

CTDs	**Cumulative trauma disorders**
CTS	**Carpal Tunnel Syndrome**
HSE	**Health Safety and Environment**
MSDs	**Musculoskeletal Disorders**
NSSA	**National Social Security Authority**
OHS	**Occupational Health and Safety**
PPE/C	**Personal Protective Equipment/ Clothing**
RSI	**Repetitive strain injuries**
RSI	**Repetitive strain injuries**
SPSS	**Statistical Package for Social Sciences**
WMSDs	**Work Related Musculoskeletal disorders**

Table of Contents

CHAPTER 1: INTRODUCTION

1.1 Background of study

Ergonomics is a science discipline which is concerned with understanding the relationship between humans and social-technical system elements (Colombini *et al*, 2000*)*. According to the International Labor Organization (2005), 160-270 million workers suffer from occupational diseases or accidents every year. The statistics of the Global Burden of diseases which has been developed by the World Health Organization (WHO), reported that muscular skeletal diseases (MSDs) contributes 37% of the disease burden which is attributable to occupational risk factors (Johnson *et al*. 2011). In the developed countries some mechanization was introduced but various studies show that the workers working in the brick manufacturing units suffer from musculoskeletal problems (Cook 1996, Chung and Kee, 2000; Trevelyan and Haslani, 2001). Pandey and Vats (2013) highlighted that the prevalence of MSDs has increased dramatically in developing countries. This might be a result of poor mechanization and poor working environment. Workers in manufacturing industries are often exposed to ergonomic challenges (Samuels, 2005). Tasks in brick making involve a very wide range of physical action from positions and postures that may not be ideal and could place workers at risk for accidents and injuries (Manoharan, *et al* 2012). In a study by Gerr, *et al* (1991) muscular skeletal disorders in manufacturing industries are caused by repetitive task, poor postures, force and manual handling.

According to Souza *et al*. (2002), manufacturing industries occupy a prominent position on the frequency and severity of accidents, especially the type of damage caused to the worker, often permanent injuries, deaths and the long period of absence from work. Studies which were conducted in India evidenced that workers in brick making industries suffer from different health problems which are caused by poor working and carrying of heavy loads (Sett and Sahu, 2008).

Beta bricks is a construction manufacturing brick making industry which is a well-recognized brand in Zimbabwe's construction sector. It is one of the largest brick producers in Zimbabwe producing 60 to 80 million brick per year thereby creating employment for many people. They are known for producing good quality and pleasing aesthetics clay bricks. Employees at Beta Holding are involve in manual work in their daily activities which include brick setting, bricking packing and brick dispatching. Manual handling work may expose the employee to different ergonomic hazard. According to Smallwood (2004) the nature of manufacturing processes presents ergonomic challenges. Safety and health monitoring programs have been implemented at Beta Holding but there is no baseline information on ergonomics hazards associated with the work therefore creating a major problem as control measure cannot be developed to ensure safety of the employees. In this way, the present study aims to assess ergonomic hazards in a brick making industries located in Harare in Mt Hampden.

1.2 Statement of the problem

High ergonomic related challenges have been faced at XY Bricks which is evidenced by workers' complaints. According to Mt Hampden clinic (2014) an average of 23 back pain problems and other different limb pains are recorded every quarter. These problems are suspected to be emerging from the work designs and the tools and equipment used in brick making industries. Safety and health monitoring program have been implemented at Beta Holding but there is no baseline information on ergonomics hazards therefore creating a major problem as control measure cannot be developed to save the employees.

1.3 Aim
  ➢ To assess the ergonomic hazards at Beta holding.

1.4 Objectives
  ➢ To determine the common ergonomic hazards at XY Bricks.
  ➢ To determine the level of awareness of XY Bricks workers on ergonomic hazards related to their work.

1.5 Research Questions
  ➢ What are the ergonomic hazards which are commonly experienced by the employees?
  ➢ What is the level awareness of XY Bricks employees on ergonomic hazard?

1.6 Justification

The recurrence of an average of 23 back and limb injuries every quarter have brought a concern to occupational safety and health performance of XY Bricks. The research will help XY Bricks to know the ergonomic hazards in workplace and to manage the identified hazards. By identifying the hazards and managing them this will protect the employees' health and safety. The study information will also bridge the gap found in Zimbabwe's ergonomic challenges baseline information relative to brick manufacturing industries. Therefore the employers in brick making

11

industries will be able to put measures that will ensure safety of the employees. The research will also give XY Bricks financial benefits as the research will help to prevent accidents and injuries that will cost the organization in compensating.

CHAPTER 2 LITERATURE REVIEW

2.1 Ergonomic Hazards at workplaces

Ergonomics is the study of workplace design, tools, environment, product, equipment, tool, environment, and system which considers human being's physical and psychological capabilities and improves the work systems of productivity and effectiveness while assuring wellbeing and workers safety and health (Fernandez and Marley 1998). According to Chapanis (1985) ergonomics determines and relates information about human abilities, limitations, behaviour and other workplace characteristics which may include design of machines, tools, jobs, the environment and the tasks to produce quality production, in a comfortable, safe manner.

Ergonomic Hazards refers to physical stressors and workplace conditions that pose a risk of injury or illness to the musculoskeletal system of the worker (NOISH 1992). They have an impact negative impact to the employees same as to the employer. If these ergonomic hazards are poor managed they may result to work related musculoskeletal disorders. Well-designed jobs improve employees' efficiency, safety, and satisfaction (Grant, 1996). If work or equipment is not suitable to the worker, the worker experiences discomfort. If the workplace is ergonomically designed the workstation will be safe and comfortable for the worker. The principle goal of ergonomics is to make the job and workplace fit for the employee not vice versa (Al swaity and Enshassi 2005). Kroemer (2002) highlighted that ergonomic hazards may include awkward postures, forceful movements, repetitive, improper postures, improper designs and equipment. Ergonomics hazards may arise from poor job designs and organizational factors which include excessive work durations, excessive work rates, external pacing of work, less time to rest and lack of task variety (Luopajarvi, 1990).

Ergonomic hazards can be classified into physical and cognitive ergonomic hazards. Physical ergonomics deals with the physical load on the human body when performing work activities. Physical ergonomics deals with human physical and bio mechanical characteristics as they interact with physical activities (Karwowski and Marras, 2003). It deals with the human body's responses to physical and physiological stress. Example of physical ergonomics hazards include; working postures, working hours, works that require a lot of force and repetitive work. Although physical risk factors are important first-line risk factors, there are other plausible factors such as organizational and psychosocial factors that may provoke a disorder or indirectly influence the

13

effect of physical risk factors (Hagberg *et al.*, 1995). Cognitive ergonomics is another class of ergonomic hazards. It is a developing class of ergonomics. It deals with human factors including their capabilities. Cognitive ergonomics emphases on the appropriate between human cognitive abilities and limitations and the machine, task, and environment, organizational hazards and environment hazards which affect workers who operate at the place of work therefore these hazardous factors can influence occupational health discomforts of workers (Grant,1996). This approach addresses problems such as attention distribution, decision making, formation of learning skills, and usability of human-computer systems, cognitive aspects of metal load, stress and human errors at work (Canas *et al.,* 2010).

2.2 Benefits of ergonomics

Ergonomics is important because it enhances worker's performance and it also prevents workers from work related injuries. It is directed towards to fit workers with their work task and jobs, equipment, environment and work systems to ensure that the workplaces are efficient, safe, and comfortable. According to Jayaratne (2012) ergonomics can solve physical, psychological and social aspects of work-related problems, thus optimizing human well-being and overall system performance. Application of ergonomics principles improves the quality of working life. The major importance of ergonomics is that it improves the workplace environment so that it best suits the workers and enables efficiency and quality production. According to Kroemer (2002) ergonomics determines human characteristics, limitations, capabilities and desires which are necessary for the workplace design, increasing human efficiency and workers' safety. The spectrum of ergonomics includes environmental factors and physical factors. It is important for the work design, work task, the environment to suit the capabilities and needs of the worker. (Purnawatt, 2007) in his study he mentioned that ergonomics is still considered a low priority as a result there is limited use of capital and low levels of enforcement.

2.3 Effects of poor ergonomics

Ergonomics should be considers in the design of workplace and the job should suit or fit the employees by any means. Lack of consideration of ergonomics in the design of workplaces and jobs can result in injuries and illness, fatigue and discomfort, inefficient working practices, poor quality of work and errors, equipment which is awkward and uncomfortable to use, lost time and poor morale. Therefore in the long run ergonomics challenges can affect the productivity of the company. Poor ergonomics can results in Work Related Musculoskeletal disorders (WMSDs).

WMSDs can be defined as any injury to the human support system, including the bones, cartilage, muscles, ligaments, tendons, blood vessels, nerves due to exposure to hazards at the workplace (Rolander, 2001). MSDs, impact negatively on worker's ability to perform tasks resulting in them being unable to maintain their quality of life (Stock *et al*, 1998). Disorders have resulted in prominent problems in industries in form of workers health problems and financial problems due to reduced worker capabilities and lessening production (Luopajarvi, 1990). In a study by Saldana (1996) MSDs may affect the body soft tissues, including damage to the tendons, tendon sheath, muscles, and nerves of the hands, wrist, elbow, shoulder, neck and back. Therefore if an organisation gives a blind eye to ergonomics principles it will lose a lot in the business long run. According to Michalak-Turcotte (2000) sufferers of WMSDs may experience numbness, tingling, pain, decreased strength or swelling of the affected area. According to Putz-Anderson (1988) the average employee loses nearly two days of work each year as a result of these disorders. However, disorders such as carpal tunnel syndrome can also be caused or aggravated by no occupational factors (Franklin *et al* 1991). Poor ergonomics can lead to health challenges that may include cumulative trauma disorders, repetitive strain injuries, carpal tunnel syndrome, tenosynovitis and tendonitis (Haupt *et al*, 2004).Below is the explanation of the health challenges.

2.3.1 Cumulative trauma disorders (CTDs).
Cumulative trauma disorders (CTD) is one of disease most common among workers in industries. CTDs includes hand and wrist repetitive trauma injuries or illnesses. According to Brogmus and Mark (1991) brick manufacturing processes in US are ranked in the top 10 of highest job classifications that incur high percentage of cumulative trauma disorders claims. CTDs can results from combination of nervous system and musculosketal disorders which can caused by improper postures, repetitive work, vibrations and forceful work exertions. CTDs are examples of Cumulative Trauma Disorders include carpal tunnel syndrome (CTS), tenosynovitis, and tendinitis

2.3.2 Repetitive strain injuries
Musculo-skeletal Disorders (MSD) in the neck, shoulders and upper limbs as well as of the lower back also referred to as repetitive strain injuries (RSIs), cause distress and disability (Baril *et al* 1994). In most cases Repetitive Strain Injuries (RSIs) results from repetitive motions, which are performed one at a time in a very short work cycle.

2.3.3 Carpal tunnel syndrome
It is a type of nerve entrapment results from the buildup of pressure on the median nerve for the construction workers due to carrying of loads and strong gripping for long time (Brogmus and

15

Marko, 1991). Cumulative trauma disorders are one the most severe disorder that is expressed by employees (Gerard, 1996). CTS can occur because of swollen tendons within the carpal tunnel area. Construction work leaves the worker at high risk of CTS. If CTS remains untreated the condition may deteriorate and may cause a loss of grip strength, increased pain during the night, and the permanent loss of hand function.

2.3.4 Tenosynovitis

Tenosynovitis is the tenderness of tendons and sheath which is related with works demanding great wrist deviation of the workers (Luopajarvi *et al.*, 1979). In general terms it can be called irritation of the synovial cover of the tendon caused by Cumulative Trauma Disorders risk factors. Poor work station designs, poor tool designs, excessive work may contribute to the development of the diseases.

2.3.5 Tendonitis

This disease occurs when a tendon is repetitively used thereby causing soreness. Repetitive or cumulative injuries like tendonitis occur commonly in jobs where a great deal of repetition occurs (Schneider *et al.*, 1999). When conducting normal work the tendons fibers can have small effects which can be healed by the body unlike excessive use and lack of recovery time does not allow the healing of the tears completely. Tendonitis is a form of tendon inflammation that occurs when a muscle or tendon is repeatedly tensed (Putz-Anderson, 1988). A form of tendon According to (Putz-Anderson, 1988) lack of proper rest and recovery time required for tissues to heal may cause permanent damage to the tendons. Tendonitis usually affects the neck, elbows, shoulders and wrists. The risk factors for tendonitis are repetition, frequency, awkward postures, vibrations and force.

2.4 Risk factors for musculoskeletal disorders

A risk factor can be defined as an attribute or exposure that increases the probability of diseases or disorder (Basra and Crawford 1995). Work related musculoskeletal disorders can be caused by the working environment, job type, and tool being used. According to Putz-Anderson (1988) risk factors results from stressors being applied to specific parts of the body during the execution of tasks. Risk factors are actions in the workplace, workplace conditions, or a combination thereof that may cause or aggravate a work related musculoskeletal disorders (Ergoweb 2008). Singh *et al* (2009) if the work demands exceeds what the physical body of the employees is capable of handling, the employee may suffer from MSD and CTD injuries. In a study by Trevelyen and Haslam (2001) it was concluded that poor standing postures and undesirable wrist position are the risk factors that may result in MSDs in brick making industry According to Gigstad (2002) there are a number of risk factors associated with the development of cumulative trauma injuries in industry. However Kostiuk (2008) highlighted that it is difficult to measure how each factor contribute to the development of MSD's because they all affect each other. Among the most prevalent of the risk factors include force, vibration, repetition, thermal stressors and postures (Putz-Anderson, 1988). Ayoub (1990) highlighted that these risk factors become hazardous due to prolonged repetitive, often in a forceful and awkward manner, without sufficient rest or recovery. In a study by Qutubuddin *et al.,* (2013) it was reviewed that workers experienced injuries in different body parts due to work process and management inaction in providing safe work environment

2.5 Management of ergonomic hazards

As much as an industry can have ergonomic hazards the hazards can be dealt with to make the workplace ergonomic hazard free (Faucet, *et al.,* 2002). Installation of ergonomic principles can improve safety and productivity and reducing employer costs (Frymoyer 1997). Ergonomic hazards can be managed by properly designing of the job or work station and selecting of the appropriate tools or equipment for that job. The interventions identified to reduce the risk of MSDs in construction could be classified as: new materials, new tools and equipment, improved work practices, improved work organization and planning, education and exercise and personal protection equipment (Bronkhorst *et al.,* 1997). According to Henry (2004) ergonomics practices can help the workplace by reorganizing, or redesigning the workstation, by allowing employees to rotate jobs, decreasing the number of repetitions required in the task, reducing the force required in the task, providing education training on correct posture for the tasks and encourage stretches during break times. Below are the ergonomics hazards controls

2.5.1 Engineering controls

Engineering controls refer to a physical modification of task, process, workstation, tools and equipment in a way that will help in preventing any harm or danger. Karwowski and Marras, (2003) engineering control can be used as an effective measure controlling the workplace hazards. They place a role in reducing the exposure of risk at the source by eliminating variables. The use of engineering controls can reduce the injury risks. Examples of engineering controls include introducing lifting mechanisms in industries, redesigning workstation layouts, reducing vibrations

17

effects by using robotic arms, changing the operation process, use of machines to reduce repetitive and awkward postures.

2.5.2 Administrative control.

These are controls which include the use of workplace policies, work procedures and practices which prevent the exposure of the employees to the ergonomics hazards by using administrative techniques such as adding number of employees to conduct a certain job, job rotation, introducing recovery breaks, training and awareness programs. Administrative controls involve changing how or when employees do their jobs, such as scheduling work and rotating employees to reduce exposure (Spellman 2006). Karwowski, & Marras, (2003) highlighted that administrative controls include reducing excessive frequency, duration, and force on the body by prohibiting overtime. Administrative controls are deemed less effective than engineering controls because they reduce the frequency and duration of risk exposure thereby not reducing the hazard directly at the source. According to Konz, (1984) Administrative controls are applied when engineering controls are either not effective or cost efficient.

2.5.3 Personal protective equipment's

The use of PPE is considered as the last priority because it does not eliminate the ergonomic hazards but it can work to reduce or minimize exposure to the hazard. According to Spellman (2006) using PPE is often essential, but it is generally the last line of defense after engineering controls, work practices and administrative controls. It is used when hazards are not controllable from the source. PPE include the use of helmets, safety shoes, gloves, goggles, earmuffs, to mention just a few and all these provide support and shield the employee from the hazard therefore reducing exposure. It is critical to ensure that introduced PPE controls fit the individual employee, are appropriate for the task, and do not contribute to extreme postures or force (Konz, 1984).

2.6 Influence of ergonomic training and awareness to employees

According to (Patkin 1987) application of ergonomics result in improved working techniques, reducing human errors and accidents and increased efficiency. Training is the acquisition of knowledge, skills, and abilities to perform more effectively (Blanchard & Thacker, 1999). Poor work ergonomics can results to slow development of diseases such as Cumulative trauma disorders, repetitive strain injuries, musculoskeletal disorders and occupational overuse syndrome. If workers are aware of work tasks and equipment that do not include ergonomic principles in their design, workers may be able to report or complain if exposed to undue physical stress, strain, and overexertion which may include vibration, awkward postures, forceful exertions, repetitive motion, and heavy lifting. According to Annis & McConville (1996) the objective of this division of ergonomics is to create the best possible job situation to enhance the worker's physical and mental health, production efficiency, and product quality. Ergonomics awareness will help in recognizing ergonomic risk factors in the workplace and it is an essential first step in correcting hazards and improving worker protection. In a study which was conducted in Malaysia by Shameem *et al.* (2001), industrial workers in Malaysia are were less educated and are ignorant of environmental and working standards, therefore they were not able to complain about work conditions. Bohr (2000) further reported that participants who received ergonomic training reported less stress and pain/discomfort than did those who had not received training.

CHAPTER THREE: RESEARCH METHODOLOGY

3.1 Description of study area

[3]XY Bricks is a brick making company established in 1953. The company traced its origin from Alpha Bricks which was later named XY Bricks in 1991 after of ownership. In 2011 the company started manufacturing concrete roofing. XY Bricks has two brick making plants which are Plant 1 and Plant 2. This research will focus on the Plant 1 brick making plant covering from brick molding up to brick dispatch. Figure 3.1 below shows the location of XY Bricks.

Figure 3.1: location map for XY Bricks.

3.2 Research Design

This study follows a cross sectional research design. Its main focus was to assess ergonomic hazard at XY Bricks. The researcher collected data in the month of August 2016. The research involved the use of questionnaires and an international hazard checklist to acquire information on the ergonomic hazards associated with the work. The research sample was drawn from five work sections covering from brick molding up to brick dispatch and these were; brick extruding, brick cutting, brick setting, brick packing and brick dispatching. A cross sectional study was conducted as the data was collected at one time at one worksite. Information on work shifts and schedules were obtained from the department supervisor.

3.3 Study Population

Beta Holding consist of two brick making plants namely Plant 1 and Plant 2, making them two work departments. The two plants consist of 200 employees in total. The departments consist of same work section namely brick extruding, brick cutting, brick setting, brick packing and brick dispatching. Below is the summarised population distribution:

Table 3.1: Research Population

Departments	Work Sections					
	Mixing	cutting	setting	packing	Dispatching	TOTAL
Plant 1	2	2	36	36	36	112
Plant 2	2	2	28	28	28	88
Total	4	4	64	64	64	200

---

[3] Due to data protection reasons this chapter has been changed by the editors.

3.4 Sample and sampling procedures

XY Bricks consist of two brick making plants namely Plant 1 and Plant 2. Thereby, making two different departments, Plant 1 department and Plant 2 department. Out of the two brick making department (Plant 1 and Plant 2) the researcher used purposive sampling to select one department (Plant 1) from which the research participants were to be selected. Plant 1 department at Beta Holding Mt Hampden was selected because it is the department which consist of high number of employees among the two departments and it is the department with high complains of body pains. Purposive sampling methods were used to choose work sections were the participants were to be chosen from and the work sections include brick extruding, brick cutting, brick setting, brick packing and brick dispatching. Strata were created using stratified random sampling to group the above mentioned work sections. From the created strata groups the researcher used convenient sampling to choose research respondents from brick extruding and brick cutting, Since 2 experts are needed per shift respectively 4 respondents were chosen. Cluster sampling technique was used to group employees from brick setting, brick packing and brick dispatching. From the selected cluster groups the researcher used random sampling to select the actual respondents to answer his research questions. The data was collected from both the shifts day shift and night shift. Below are the summarized sample sizes.

3.5 Data Collection Methods and Techniques

This research was based on primary data through the use of questionnaires and NIOSH inspection checklist for ergonomic factors as methods of gathering the required data.

3.5.1 Questionnaires

Semi structured questionnaires were used to determine ergonomic hazards experienced by employees and to assess if the employees were aware of ergonomic hazards. The questionnaire consisted of closed and open-ended questions. Questionnaires were designed to suit all work sections. The questionnaires were handed over physically to respondents. Out of the 40 administered questionnaires there were 38 respondents and 2 uncertainties. Table 3.3 below shows how the questionnaires were distributed.

Table 3.3 Questionnaire Distribution

Department Section	Number of questionnaires respondents	
	1st Shift	2nd Shift
Extruder mixer	1	1
Brick cutter	1	1
Brick setters	6	6
Brick packing	5	6
Final product dispatch	5	6
Total	18	20

The questionnaire responses were coded and tallied question-by-question to aid data presentation in Chapter four. The questionnaires were issued to respondents on the beginning of the work shift and were returned at the end of the work shift so as to avoid them from getting lost. Questionnaires were chosen because they are relatively cheap, easy to administer. This eliminated bias as information is provided in the absence of the researcher. Self-completion of questionnaires also guaranteed confidentiality. Furthermore, with closed questions, answers are standardized and this help in interpreting response.

3.5.2 NIOSH inspection checklist for ergonomic factors
The researcher conducted the inspections, observing same 40 participants which were selected as the research sample while they were doing their daily jobs. The inspections were conducted so as to assess ergonomic hazards that are experienced by the employees. The employees were observed doing a complete job cycle while the observer was paying special attention to ergonomic hazards which were on the checklist. Inspection checklist was used to note down all ergonomic hazards experienced by each work.

3.6 Data Analysis
The data obtained from the questionnaire was gathered, coded and stored into SPSS version. The information collected were presented in tables. Statistical Package for Social Sciences version 16 (SPSS) was used for descriptive analysis utilising the crosstabs tool. The tool was used to obtain the frequency and the percentiles.

CHAPTER FOUR: RESULTS

4.1 Common ergonomic hazards at XY Bricks

The results shows that the common ergonomic hazards at XY Bricks include repetition and awkward postures, forceful motions, stationary positions, vibration, tasks that externally paced and work stress. From the results all of respondents from Green brick cutter, Green brick setter and final brick dispatcher experience repeated forceful work followed by 91.6% of Green brick packers who also experience repeated forceful work hazards Findings indicate that employees from extruder mixer controller were not exposed to the hazards. The results show that generally majority of workers (green brick cutter, green brick packer, green brick setter and final brick dispatcher) were exposed of awkward postures particularly bending or leaning forward as well as lifting below knee level. The extruder mixer controller are not exposed to standing in one position for long time while all respondents from green brick cutter, green brick packer, green brick setter and final brick dispatcher are working in one position for long period. All of workers on the mixer controller are exposed to vibration hazards whilst other workers are not exposed to vibration equipment. Piece work is used as production incentive for all the employees. The results indicate that all the extruder mixer controller has sufficient work breaks and the rest of the employees have insufficient work breaks. (*see appendix 3*).

Generally all mixer controllers are not exposed to work that is externally pace while all the other respondents from Green brick cutter, green brick setter, green brick packing and final brick dispatch are doing work that is externally paced. All extruder mixer controllers are not exerting force with hands while all of respondents from Brick cutter, brick setting and brick packing exerting force with their hands. The results shows that 90.9% of the participants from green brick packing and all participants from the mixer extruder uses of tools or handles. All of participants from extruder mixer controllers, brick cutter, green brick setters, green brick packing and final brick dispatch are standing continuously for more than 30 minutes while performing their daily jobs and no employees from brick cutter are standing continuously for more than 30 minutes while performing their daily jobs. All of participants from the green brick cutter are sitting for more than 30 minutes without standing or moving around and participants from mixer controllers, brick cutter, green brick setters, green brick packing and final brick dispatch show that they are not sitting for more than 30 minutes without standing or moving around. Generally all green brick packers and final brick dispatch participants perform their duties kneeling. Among all employees from all work sections, 90.9% participants from green brick packer only are performing work with hands raised above shoulder heights. From the results is evidenced that all of respondents from brick cutter, brick setter, brick packer and final brick dispatch are performing work while bending and twisting the wrist. All green brick setter and final brick dispatch participants and 81.8% of green brick packing participants are lowering objects more than twice per minute for more than 15 minutes. From the results it is evidenced that all of respondents from green brick packing and final brick dispatch are lifting and lowering objects between floor and waist shoulder height when doing work. All work sections are lifting objects that cannot be held close to the body. Results shows that all of respondents from green brick packing are lifting lowering or carry objects weighing more than 22.6 kilograms. (*see appendix 4*)

4.2 The level of awareness of XY Bricks workers on ergonomic hazards

Majority of the respondents, 63% are not aware what ergonomic hazards are and 37% of the respondents are aware of what ergonomic hazards. Of the remaining 37% of the respondents 13.2% workers are aware of awkward, 8.1% of the respondents are aware of forceful work and 5.3% of the respondents are aware of work stressors. Table 4.4 below shows the results

Fig 4.2 The Knowledge of respondents on ergonomic hazards (n=38)

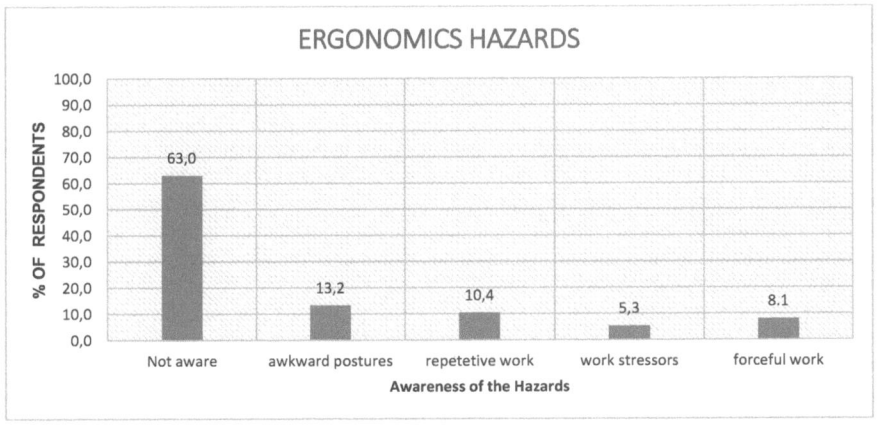

24

CHAPTER 5: DISCUSSION

5.1 Common Ergonomic hazards at Beta Holding

The ergonomics hazards which were identified included repetition, forceful motions, stationary positions, vibration, tasks that externally paced and work stress. Below is the discussion of the ergonomic hazards.

Generally, the highest percentage of respondents having repeated forceful work is faced by employees from green brick cutting, green brick setting, green brick packing and brick dispatch work this might be due to the high speed of the machine which moves at a fast speed so as to meet daily targets and due to manual work. Forceful work is inherent of industries that involve manual labour (Scott 2009)

All the employees from all the work sections use same body part repeatedly when they are conducting their daily jobs this might be due to the nature and design of the job that require repeated work and these might be due to poor technological advancements. Job design where employees perform single main task in the brick making process can lead to repetitive activities (Ndivhudzannyi 2003). While green brick setters are exposed to bending this might be due to poor chairs they use while working which does not have a back and hand rests. Green brick setting, green brick packing and brick dispatch might be exposed to bending due to the level of the conveyor belts which is below the waist level, the low level of the brick firing clamps bases. Bending might be an attribute of poor lifting techniques that are adopted by the employees. The mainly cause of repeated bending and twisting of the trunk is work station design and position of equipment and tools (Kumar, 2001).

Respondent from green brick setters, green brick packing and brick dispatching highlighted that they are kneeling when working. This might be due position of the conveyor belt they try to reach brick from thereby forcing them to kneel. Awkward kneeling at work is caused by interactions between the operators and machines or materials in the production system (Peterson, 1997). Green brick packing and final brick dispatching respectively are perform work with hands raised above shoulder heights. This could be due to high level of brick stacks were they pack and unpack bricks. The position of the bricks might be forcing them to raise their hands so as to reach the bricks. Worker' physical capabilities maybe affected by work designs and work equipment (Chung and Kee, 2000).

Green brick cutting, green brick setting, green brick packing and final brick dispatching perform work while bending and twisting at the wrist. This might be due to the position of bricks and the design of the tools they use when conducting work. Respondents from mixer controlling, green brick setting, green brick packing and final brick dispatch stand continuously for more than 30 minutes when conducting their daily duties. Thereby exposing them to poor postures this might be due to position of parts and equipment they use, speed of task that does not allow the employees to change the body position and this could also be due to duration of the task that are done continuously without giving the body chance to change its position. Work operators are forced to adopt certain position because corporate standards for human needs were not implemented fully and used in designing of the work processes (Wulff et al., 2000). The respondents from the brick cutter show that 0% of them are standing for more than 30 minutes this might be due to the nature of their job which is done while sitting.

The results show that the respondents from brick packing are lifting, pushing, or pulling more than 22.6kgs which is against the NOISH standards regulation. This might be due to absents of proper machinery which can be used to move the bricks from the conveyor belt to the firing clamps and the pace of work cycle. Lifting, lower or carry objects weighing more than 22.6kgs this might be due to the need to meet their targets and the high level of target that are unrealistic to meet forcing them to overload themselves This is agreed in a study by Pandey and Vats (2013) were it was highlighted that manual handling of bricks expose employees to objects weighing more than 50lb (22.6kgs). In a study by Mukhopadhyay (2008) his results showed that brick making employees were paid for the number of units of bricks produced, resulting to a tendency to working for longer working hours and over exhausting of workers

It is evidenced by the results that respondents from green brick cutter, green brick setters, green brick packing and final brick dispatch are exerting force with hands while carrying their duties this could be due to strength and effort required by the job. This is supported in a study by (Pandey and Vats, 2013) where he found that male and female workers in brick industry usually require exerting force with their hands. Respondents from mixer controller are not exerting force this is due to the nature of their job that does not require strength to perform the require task as they only operate automatic machines. Employees from green brick cutter, green brick setters, brick packing and brick dispatch are lifting more than 2.7 with one hand which against NOISH standards regulations. This could be due to the work load which forces them to carry two or more bricks at the same time so as to cover the daily work targets. Daily targets influence fast working pace, where most workers lift more than two bricks (Ndivhudzannyi, 2003). While employees from green brick setting and final brick dispatching and green brick packing are lifting or lowering objects more than once per minute for continuous period of more than 15 minutes. This might be due to speed of work or work cycle and frequency of work. The employees might be forced to lift or lower objects continuous due to high production targets that need to be meet. Bao *et al.,* (1997) highlighted that well balanced production system with less production workers result in high body movements

Respondents from green brick cutter, green brick setting, green brick packing and brick dispatch shows that they are working in one position for long periods. This could be due to the nature of the job which is stationary and absence of job rotation and work pressure which does not allow the employees to rest or to change the working position. Work designs is the major contribution of static postures that may result in development problems of shoulder and upper limbs (Buckle and Stubbs, 1990). The results shows that workers from green brick setting, green brick packing and brick dispatch are standing for long periods while working. This could be due to the nature of the job which is stationary and absence of job rotation and work pressure which does not allow the employees to sit down. This could also be an attribute of the nature of the job which forces the employees to conduct work while standing. The design of the work system provides a number of performance constraints which the operator should perform within the assigned parameters (Neumann 2004). While respondents from green brick cutter shows that they are working while in sitting position for long periods. This could be due to the nature of the job were equipment which

26

are used should be operated while one is sitting and absence of job rotation and work pressure which does not allow the employees to rest or to change the working position. The nature of the job itself primarily determines the worker's mechanical exposure profile (Allread *et al.*, 2000).

Vibration, environment and work stress are also other common ergonomic hazards. The results shows that the mixer controller are using vibrating hand tools. This could be due to the design of the tool which vibrates when working. This is augmented by Palmer, *et al,* (2006) and Griffin (2006) who reported that vibration exposure can be related to the types of work processes and types of tools used. Green brick packer and final brick dispatch respectively use of hand to tools or handle parts thereby posing a hazard to the employees. This might be due to the design of parts, equipment or tools which need to be handled by the employees. According to Hagberg *et al.,* (1995) poor designed tools and handles may be the cause of direct mechanical pressure on the body. The results also shows that respondents from mixer control, green brick cutter and green brick setting are not using any tool or handle due to their nature of work.

Piece work for all work sections is used as production incentive for all work sections. This could be an attribute of high production target set by the organization. The results shows that there is insufficient work breaks for green brick setting, green brick packing and brick dispatch. This might because of work pressure to meet set production targets and also pressure to earn production incentives. A study by Ndivhudzannyi (2003) the daily targets encourages the missing of breaks. Sufficient work breaks at the mixer controller this could be due to the type of machine which is automated that can allow the employees to take a break. According to Basra and Crawford (1995) piece work system arise from high production needs by the employer.

The results shows that respondents from the task from mixer controller are not externally paced this might be due to the reason that they are the ones who control the brick production machine. It is also evidence that respondents from brick cutter, brick setter, brick packing and final brick dispatch are having tasks that are externally paced this could be due to production targets and the procedure which does not allow the machine to be stopped so as to meet the set targets. Brick sorters mainly experience excessive work encouraging then to adopt high working pace than necessary (Ndivhudzannyi, 2003). This is supported by Putz-Anderson (1988) who reported that ergonomic problems can be caused by production demand and fault work methods.

5.2 Ergonomic hazard awareness
The results show that the majority of the employees were not aware of the ergonomic hazards. This could be due to little or no knowledge on safety and health issues. Low level of ergonomics awareness could be due to the fact that the employees did not receive any training on ergonomics during the induction period. This is agreed in a study by Shameem *et al.* (2001); Malaysian industrial workers experienced less work freedom because most of them were not educated and were not aware of the safe work environmental standards. This agrees with Koradecka (2001) who stated highlighted that about one billion employees work without receiving ergonomics awareness.

13.2% of the respondents were aware of awkward postures. This could be due to the nature of their jobs which make them deviate from the neutral posture most working hours of the day.
10.4% of the identified repetitive work. This could be due to their work tasks that have small

27

work circle which require to be done continuously. Some of the respondents identified work stressors this could be due to piece work they are exposed to when working. 8% of the respondents identified forceful work as hazards associated with their work tasks. This might be due to muscle pains they experience. In a study by Mukwazhe and Gwisai (2016) it was highlighted that hazards are identified because of manual tasks that are conducted daily.

CHAPTER 6 CONCLUSIONS AND RECOMMENDATIONS

6.1 Conclusions

From the study findings it is concluded employees from Beta Bricks commonly experience ergonomic hazards such repetition, awkward postures, forceful motions, stationary working positions, vibration, work stress. The ergonomic hazards experienced vary with work station and this can be attributed to poor work design, work cycle time, duration of task, production pressure, poor equipment. The findings show that majority of employees lack ergonomic hazards awareness.

6.2 Recommendations

From the study results it can be recommended that there is need to use engineering controls by redesign the workplace, tools and equipment. The company should also use administrative controls through the use of preventive programs and conducting of trainings on ergonomic so that employees will be aware of ergonomic hazards and ergonomic hazards control measures for example training on lifting techniques. This will help to minimize the ergonomic risk factors in the workplace and this may improve health of the employees and improve productivity.

The study revealed that the majority employees are not aware of the ergonomic hazards associated with their work tasks. The researcher therefore recommends awareness training to be conducted at all levels so as to increase employees' knowledge on ergonomic hazards.

The organization should also encourage job rotation so that workers will have enough time to rest and this will help exposure time to the ergonomic hazards.

References

Allread, W. G., Marras, W. S., and Burr, D. L. (2000). Measuring trunk motions in industry: variability due to task factors, individual differences, and the amount of data collected Ergonomics, 43(6), 691-701

Annis, J. F., and McConville, J. (1996). Anthropometry. *occupational safety and health-New York, 27,* 1-46.

Ayoub, M, A. (1990). Ergonomic Deficiencies: Pain at Work, journal of occupational medicine, 32,52-57.

Bao, S., Winkel, J., Mathiassen, S. E., and Shahnavaz, H. (1997). Interactive effect of ergonomics and production engineering on shoulder-neck exposure - a case study of assembly work in China and Sweden. International Journal of Industrial Ergonomics, 20, 75- 85.

Baril, R., and IRSST (Québec). (1994). Étude exploratoire des processus de réinsertion sociale et professionnelle des travailleurs en réadaptation. [Québec]: IRSST.

Basra, G, and Crawford, J. O., (1995). Contemporary Ergonomics. Assessing work-related upper limb disorders in a brick making factory. 480-485.

Blanchard, P. N., and Thacker, J. W. (1999). Effective training: Strategies, systems, and practices.

Bohr PC. (2000). Efficacy of office ergonomics education. Journal of Occupational Rehabilitation, 10:243-55.

Brogmus, G. E., and Marko, R. (1991). Cumulative trauma disorders of the upper extremities: the magnitude of the problem in US industry. *Advances in industrial ergonomics and safety III. London, UK: Taylor & Francis,* 95-102.

Buckle, P. W., and Stubbs, D. A. (1990). Epidemiological aspects of musculoskeletal disorders of the shoulder and upper limbs. *Contemporary ergonomics. London, UK: Taylor & Francis,* 75-8.

Bullock, M.J. (Ed.), Ergonomic: The physiotherapist in the workplace.*Edinburgh London Melbourne and New York.*51-78.

Canas, J. Di Stasi, L. L., Renner, R., Staehr, P., Helmert, J. R., Velichkovsky, B. M., & Pannasch, S. (2010). Saccadic peak velocity sensitivity to variations in mental workload. *Aviation, Space, and Environmental Medicine, 81*(4), 413-417.

Chapanis, A. (1985). Some reflections on progress. In *Proceedings of the Human Factors Society Annual Meeting.* Sage CA: Los Angeles, CA: SAGE Publications 9(1), 1-8

Chung, M. K., & Kee, D. (2000). Evaluation of lifting tasks frequently performed during fire brick manufacturing processes using NIOSH lifting equations. *International Journal of Industrial Ergonomics, 25*(4), 423-433.

Colombini, D., Occhipinti, E., Molteni, G., & Grieco, A. (2000). Evaluation of work chairs. *International Encyclopedia of Ergonomics and Human Factors, 3*, 921.

Cook, T. M., Rosecrance, J. C., & Zimmermann, C. L. (1996). Work-related musculoskeletal disorders in bricklaying: a symptom and job factors survey and guidelines for improvements. *Applied occupational and environmental hygiene, 11*(11), 1335-1339.

Faucet, J., Garry, M., Nadler, D., and Ettare, D. 2002, A test of two training interventions to prevent Work-related Musculoskeletal Disorders of the upper extremity. Applied Ergonomics 33, 337-347

Fernandez, IE. and Marley, R.M., Applied Occupational Ergonomics: A Textbook, Kendall-Hunt Publishing, 1998.

Franklin,G.M., Haug,J., Heyer,N., Checkoway,H. and Peck,N. (1991). Occupational carpal tunnel syndrome in Washington State, 1984-1988. American Journal of Public Health, 81, (6), 741-746.

Frymoyer, J. 1997, Cost and control of industrial Musculoskeletal Disorders of the workplace: principles and practice. St. Louis, Missouri: Mosby-Year Book, INC. PP.62-71.

Gerald, M. (1996). Effects of key stiffness on force and the development of fatigue while typing. American Industrial Hygiene Association Journal 57, 849-854

Gerr, F., Letz, R., & Landrigan, P. J. (1991). Upper-extremity musculoskeletal disorders of occupational origin. *Annual review of public health, 12*(1), 543-566.

Grant, R. M. (1996). Prospering in dynamically-competitive environments: Organizational capability as knowledge integration. *Organization science, 7*(4), 375-387.

Griffin, M. J. (2007). Discomfort from feeling vehicle vibration. *Vehicle System Dynamics, 45*(7-8), 679-698.

Hagberg, M., Silverstein, B., Wells, R., Smith, M. J., Hendrick, H. W., Carayon, P., & Perusse, M. (1995). Identification, measurement and evaluation of risk. *Work Related Musculoskeletal Disorders (WMSD's), a reference book for prevention. Taylor & Francis, London*, 139-145.

Haupt, T. C., Deacon, C., & Smallwood, J. (2005). Importance of healthy older construction workers. *Acta Structilia: Journal for the Physical and Development Sciences, 12*(1), 1-19.

Haupt T. C., Smallwood, J., (2005), Rethinking and Revitalizing Construction Safety, health, Environment and Quality. cm W99 Working Commission. 'The Proceedings of the W99 Triennial International Council for Research and Innovation in Building and Construction' (Cm). CREATE, Port Elizabeth. 2005. ISBN 0-620-33919-5.

Henry. J. T. (2004). A Study of psychosocial work factors and ergonomic risk factors and how they affect worker stress and musculoskeletal discomfot in assembly workers within a manufacturing industry environment.

Jayaratne, K. (2012). Ergonomic considerations in school environments-the need for widening the scope. *Work, 41*(Supplement 1), 5543-5546.

Johnson, A., and Widyanti, A. (2011). Cultural influences on the measurement of subjective mental workload. *Ergonomics, 54*(6), 509-518.

Karwowski, W., and Marras, W. S. (Eds.). (2003). *Occupational ergonomics: engineering and administrative controls.* CRC Press.

Konz, S. A. (1984) Work Design: Industrial Ergonomics. John Wiley and Sons Canada, Limited, New York.2,614.

Koradecka, D., and Golebiowska, A. (2001). Biosketch: Wojciech Bogumil Jastrzebowski. *International Encyclopedia of Ergonomics and Human Factors*, 21.

Kumar, S. (2001). Theories of musculoskeletal injury causation. Ergonomics, 44, 17– 47

Luopajarvi, T. (1990). Ergonomic analysis of workplace and postural load. *Ergonomics: the physiotherapist in the workplace. Edinburgh, London, Melbourne and New York*, 51-78.

Manoharan, P. K., Jha, S. K., & Singh, B. K. (2012). Modeling the risk factors in ergonomic processes in Brick kilns workers using Fuzzy Logic. *International Journal of Applied Science and Engineering Research, 1*(1), 92-97.

Michalak-Turcotte, C. (2000) Controlling dental hygiene work-related musculoskeletal disorders: The ergonomic process. Journal of Dental Hygiene, 74, 41-48.

Mufamadi Ndivhudzannyi, E. (2003). The study of work-related musculoskeletal disorders amongst workers in brick making factory in South Africa.

Mukhopadhyay, P. (2008). Risk factors in manual brick manufacturing in India. *HFESA J Ergon Aus, 22*, 6-25.

Mukwazhe, L and Gwisai R. (2016). Ergonomic hazard risk assessment in small to medium enterprises of Kadoma, Zimbabwe *2(4), 21-35*

Neumann. P. W. (2004) Identifying and monaging Risk in the design of high performance work system.

Putz-Anderson, V., & Waters, T. R. (1991, April). Revisions in NIOSH guide to manual lifting. In *national conference entitled "A national strategy for occupational musculoskeletal injury prevention—Implementation issues and research needs." Ann Arbor, MI, University of lvlichigan.*

32

NIOSH [1996]. Back belts: do they prevent injury? Cincinnati, OH: U.S. Department of

NIOSH. 1997. "Musculoskeletal Disorders in the Workplace" *Occupational Health Report Publication* No. 97-141. Dept. of Health and Human Services, Cincinnati.

Palmer, A., Qianjin, Y., & Fengwei, G. (2010). Ice-induced vibrations and scaling. *Cold Regions Science and Technology*, *60*(3), 189-192.

Pandey, K., & Vats, A. (2013). Ergonomic hazard identification of workers engaged in brick making factories. *Journal of Applied and Natural Science*, *5*(2), 297-301.

Patkin, R. A. (1987). Arbitration of Extraterritorial Discovery Disputes Between the Securities and Exchange Commission and a Foreign Broker-Dealer: A New Approach to the Restatement Balancing Test. *BU Int'l LJ*, *5*, 413.

Peterson, N. F. (1997). "Production system and individual mechanical exposure," Lic.Eng., Lund University, Lund. ISBN ISSN 1104-1080

Prevention, National Institute for Occupational Safety and Health, DHHS (NIOSH) Publication No. 94–127.

Purnawatt, S. (2007). Occupational health and safety-ergonomics improvement as a corporate responsibility of a Bali handicraft company: A case study. J. Human Ergo 36: 75-80

Putz-Anderson, V., 1988. Cumulative Trauma Disorders: a Manual for Musculoskeletal Diseases of the Upper Limbs. Taylor & Francis, London.

Rolander B, Bellner A.(2001). Experience of musculo-skeletal disorders, intensity of pain, and general conditions in work. The case of employees in non-private dental clinics in a county in southern Sweden. 65-73.

Saldana, N. 1996. Active Surveillance of Work-related Musculoskeletal Disorders: an essential component in ergonomic problems. In Bhattacharya, A. and McGlothlin, J. (Eds.), *Occupational Ergonomics: Theory and practice*. New York: Marcel Dekker. 489-500.

Saunders .M, Lewis .P and Thornhill .A (2009), Research Methods for Business Students- fifth edition, Prentice Hall, New York

Schneider, S. P (1999). Ergonomics in the construction Industry.

Scott, P. A. (Ed.). (2009). Ergonomics in developing regions: Needs and applications. CRC Press.

Sett, M. and Sahu, S. (2008) Ergonomics study on female workers in manual brick manufacturing units in West Bengal, India. Asian-Pacific Newsletter on Occupational Health and safety, 15(3), 59-60.

Shameem, S., Z. Taha, I. Nazaruddin, R.A. Ghazilla and N. Yusof, 2001. Perception and attitude of Malaysian industrial workers towards their workplace. Proceedings of the Malaysian

Ergonomics 2001: Safe and Healthy Workplaces for Better Productivity and Efficiency, Apr. 17-18, Intel Technology Sdn. Bhd., Penang.

Singh, D, Park W, and Levy, M, S. (2009) Obesity does not reduce maximum acceptable weights of lift. Applied Ergonimics,40, 1-7.

Smallwood, John, 2004. The Role of Optimum Health and Safety (H&S) in Construction Markerting.

Spellman, F. R. (2006). *Industrial Hygiene Simplified: A Guide to Anticipation, Recognition, Evaluation, and Control of Workplace Hazards.* Government Institutes.

Stock R, Stone N, Tabert A (1998) A dose-response study for 1-125 prostate implant

Trevelyan, F. C., & Haslam, R. A. (2001). Musculoskeletal disorders in a handmade brick manufacturing plant. *International Journal of Industrial Ergonomics, 27*(1), 43-55.

Wulff, I. A., Rasmussen, B., and Westgaard, R. H. (2000). Documentation in large- scale engineering design: information processing and defensive mechanisms to generate information overload. International Journal of Industrial Ergonomics, 25, 295-310

Appendixes

Appendix 1 Sample Inspection Checklist form

INSPECTION CHECKLIST FOR ERGONOMIC RISK FACTORS

Date: …................ Time: ……………... CHECKLIST NUMBER: ……….

Job title: …………………… Task: ……………………………..

Task description: …………………………………..

RISK FACTORS	YES	NO	CAUSE/DESCRIPTION
Repetition			
Repeated forceful or awkward motions			
Little or no rest			
Using same body part repeatedly			
Awkward Posture			
Bending or leaning forward			
Reaching or lifting below knee level			
Twisting or bending to the side			
Reaching above chest level			
Bending wrist frequently			
Twisting hands or forearms			
Raising arms to side or forward			
Bending neck			
Forceful Motion			
Lifting, pushing, or pulling more than 50 pounds			
Lifting more than six pounds with one hand			
Forceful gripping of material or tools			
Handling tools or material in pinch grip			
Stationary Position			
Working in one position for long periods			
Standing for long periods			
Sitting for long periods			
Direct Pressure			

Tool or equipment pressing on hand or body			
Seat or table pressing on leg or body			
Vibration			
Using vibrating hand tools			
Operating vibrating heavy equipment			
Environment			
Workplace poorly lit			
Walkways obstructed or slippery			
Work stress			
Pace of work is machine-controlled			
Piece work is used as production incentive			
Insufficient work breaks			
Poor supervision			

Inspection checklist was adapted from: NIOSH "Elements of Ergonomics Program," www.cdc.gov/niosh/eptbtr5a.html, and "Working Without Pain Train the Trainer Program," Hunter College Center for Occupational and Environmental Health.

Appendix 2: Sample Questionnaire:

QUESTIONNAIRE

TOPIC: AN ASSESSMENT OF ERGONOMIC HAZARDS IN BRICK MAKING INDUSTRY.
CASE STUDY XY BRICKS

My name is Leon Kandoko, a student from Bindura University of Science Education. I am currently studying towards degree of Bachelor of Environmental Sciences honours in Safety, Health and Environmental Management. I am carrying out study to identify of ergonomic hazards in brick making industry (XY Bricks). I am therefore requesting your assistance to participate in this survey as you associated with the work on a daily basis. I assure you of utmost confidentiality and a pledge that all the information gathered will be strictly used for academic purposes.

May you please tick and or where appropriate

QUESTIONNAIRE No…..………….

Date ……/…….. /……

1. What is your occupation?
   ……………………………………………………………………...

2. In which year did you start working in brick making industry? ……………………

3. Do you perform tasks that are externally paced? YES ☐ NO ☐

4. Do you require exerting force with your hands (gripping, pulling, and pinching)?

   YES ☐ NO ☐

5. Do you use hand tools or handle parts or objects? YES ☐ NO ☐

6. Do you stand continuously for more than 30 minutes? YES ☐ NO ☐

7. Do you sit for period of more than 30 minutes, without the opportunity to stand or move around freely? YES ☐ NO ☐

8. Do you kneel when working (one or both knees)? YES ☐ NO ☐

9. Do perform activities with hand raised above shoulder heights? YES ☐ NO ☐

10. Do you perform work while bending or twisting at the wrist? YES☐ NO☐

11. Do you worker lift or lower objects between floor and waist height or shoulder?
YES☐ NO☐

12. Do you lift or lower objects more than once per minute for continuous period of more tha15
minutes? YES☐ NO☐

13. Do you lift, lower or carry large objects that cannot be held close to the body?
YES☐ NO☐

14. Do you loft lower or carry objects weighing more than 22.6kgs? YES☐ NO☐

15. Do you know what ergonomic hazards are? YES☐ NO☐

16. If the answer in [4] is yes, state the ergonomic hazards associated with your
operations...
....
....
....

17. What measures did you put in place to reduce ergonomic hazards please specify below?
....
....

18. Do you follow any safety, health and environmental standards? YES☐ NO☐

19. Any other comments/recommendations
....
....

Thank you for taking time to assist in this survey

Appendix 3: Common ergonomic hazards at XY Bricks from Checklist

RISK FACTORS	Brick extruder % exposed	Brick cutting % exposed	Brick setting % exposed	Brick packing % exposed	Final brick dispatch % exposed
Repetition					
Repeated forceful or awkward motions	0	100	100	91.6	100
Little or no rest	0	100	100	100	100
Using same body part repeatedly	2	100	100	100	100
Awkward Posture					
Bending or leaning forward	0	100	100	100	100
Reaching or lifting below knee level	0	100	0	66	100
Twisting or bending to the side	100	100	100	100	100
Reaching above chest level	0	0	0	100	100
Bending wrist frequently	0	100	100	100	100
Twisting hands or forearms	0	0	0	0	0
Raising arms to side or forward	0	100	100	100	100
Bending neck	100	100	100	100	100
Vibration					
Using vibrating hand tools	100	0	0	0	0
Operating vibrating heavy equipment	0	0	0	0	0
Environment					
Workplace poorly lit	0	0	0	0	0
Walkways obstructed or slippery	0	0	58.3	75	83.3
Work stress					
Pace of work is machine-controlled	100	100	100	66.6	0

Piece work is used as production incentive	100	100	100	100	100
Insufficient work breaks	0	1000	100	100	100
Poor supervision	0	0	0	0	0
Forceful Motion					
Lifting, pushing, or pulling more than 22.6kgs	0	0	0	100	0
Lifting more than 2.7 with one hand	0	100	100	100	100
Forceful gripping of material or tools	0	100	100	100	100
Handling tools or material in pinch grip	0	100	100	100	100
Stationary Position					
Working in one position for long periods	0	100	100	100	100
Standing for long periods	100	0	100	100	100
Sitting for long periods	0	100	0	0	0
Direct Pressure	0	0	0	0	0
Tool or equipment pressing on hand or body	0	100	100	100	100

Exposed percentages (exposed %) represent percentage of employees who were exposed to a stated hazard.

Appendix 4: Common ergonomic hazards at XY Bricks from the Questionnaire

RISK FACTORS	Brick extruder	Brick cutting	Brick setting	Brick packing	Final brick dispatch
	% exposed	% exposed	% exposed	% exposed	% exposed
Task Externally Paced	0	100	100	100	100
Exerting force with hands	0	100	100	100	100
Use of tools or handles	2	100	100	100	84
Standing continuously for more than 30 minutes	100	0	100	90.9	72.7
Sitting for more than 30 minutes without standing or moving around	0	100	0	0	0
Kneeling when working	0	0	0	0	0
Performing work with hands raised above shoulder heights	0	0	17	90,9	100
Performing work while bending and twisting the wrist	0	100	84	90.9	100
Lowering objects more than twice per minute for more than 15 minutes	0	0	100	100	100
Lifting and lowering objects between floor and waist shoulder height	0	0	0	84	72.7
Lifting objects that cannot be held close to the body	0	0	84	100	100
Lifting lowering or carry objects weighing more than 22.6 kilograms	0	0	0	100	100

Exposed percentages(exposed %) represent percentage of employees who were exposed to a stated hazard.

YOUR KNOWLEDGE HAS VALUE

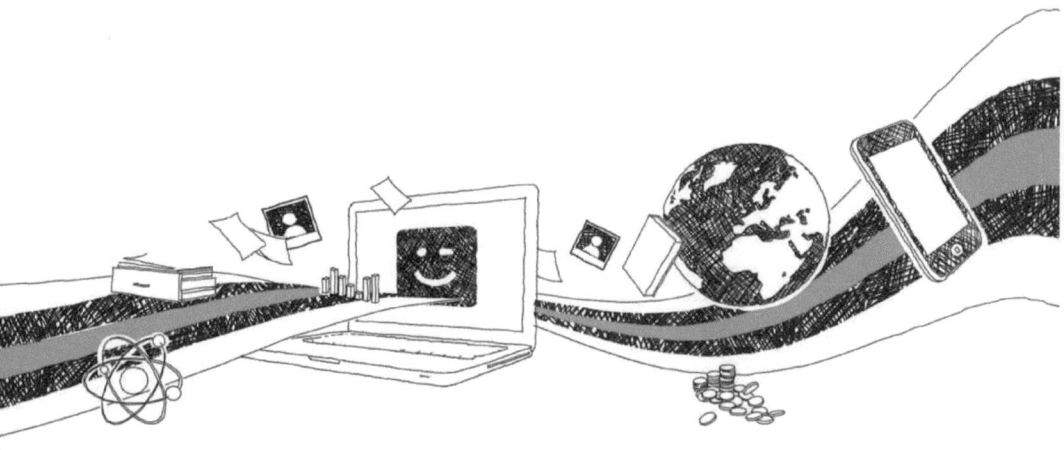

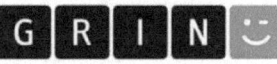